The Complete 7 Day Anti Inflammatory Diet Recipes Cookbook Easy Reduce Inflammation Plan

Your Guide to Eating to Minimize Inflammation and Maximize Health

Anti-Inflammatory Diet

Charlie Mason

CONTENTS

1 Introduction   4

2 **Chapter 1: 7-Day Meal Plan**   Pg 5

3 **Chapter 2: Five Fantastic BONUS Recipes**   Pg 27

4 **Conclusion**   Pg 32

5 **Index for Recipes**   Pg 33

As a way of saying thank you for purchasing my book, please use your link below to claim your 3 FREE Cookbooks on Health, Fitness & Dieting Instantly

https://bit.ly/2NMfuF5

You can also share your link with your friends and families whom you think that can benefit from the cookbooks or you can forward them the link as a gift!

INTRODUCTION

Most people don't think of their bodies as a battleground, but every day your body's systems are waging a war to keep you healthy. Micro armies are standing by to attack at the least provocation. When injury or illness threatens, those armies are mobilized. The result is inflammation. In the case of a cold, cut or broken bone, the response is acute and limited. However, there are many issues that lead those armies to engage not just in a battle but in an unceasing, unnecessary war.

Several disease states keep the body in a state of constant warfare. Diseases like asthma, COPD, heart disease, arthritis, diabetes, and many autoimmune diseases like Chrone's, lupus, or IBS all contribute to chronic inflammation. Conditions like obesity, stress, lack of exercise, sedentary lifestyle, smoking, or a diet of processed foods also cause the body to produce inflammation-causing hormones. This constant state of inflammation leads to an imbalance in your body. Your cells don't function efficiently, and you feel the worse for it. Aching joints, exhaustion, abdominal pain/cramps, nausea, and depressed mood are all symptoms of chronic inflammation.

One of the best ways to beat chronic inflammation is to change your diet. In the following pages, you will find an entire week's meal plan and 5 fantastic bonus recipes. While changing your diet is critical to decreasing inflammation, there are many other steps you can take. Exercise is another fantastic way to decrease inflammation by increasing your circulation and the lubrication in your joints. Light, low impact exercises like walking, swimming, or yoga is critical to achieving overall good health.

There are plenty of books on this subject on the market, thanks again for choosing this one! Every effort was made to ensure it is full of as much useful information as possible, please enjoy!

CHAPTER 1: 7-DAY MEAL PLAN

Stocking the Pantry:

Each day has a shopping list provided. There are many common pantry ingredients that you need to stock up on as you begin your anti-inflammatory diet! You'll find these throughout this book. Keeping a stocked pantry is important in sticking to any diet plan.

Spices:

- Turmeric
- Cumin
- Nutmeg
- Cinnamon
- Ginger (ground and fresh)
- Garlic (fresh)
- Sea Salt
- Pepper- black/cayenne/crushed red flakes

Grains/baking staples

- Quinoa
- Rolled/steel-cut oats
- Brown/wild rice
- Almond flour
- Coconut flour
- Baking powder
- Whole grain bread or crackers

Sauces/ cooking fats

- Olive oil
- Coconut oil
- Mirin (Japanese cooking wine)
- Soy sauce

- Tahini
- Nut butter (your choice)
- Apple cider vinegar
- Vanilla extract
- Coconut milk

Sweeteners

- Raw honey
- Blackstrap molasses

Add-ins and extras

- Chia/flax seeds
- Dried fruit
- Nuts: almonds; cashews; walnuts; pine nuts (your choice)

Day 1
Shopping list for the day:

- Chickpeas
- Parsley
- Chickpea flour
- Potato starch
- Onion
- Leafy greens
- Avocado
- Eggs
- Fresh Basil
- Melon or fruit of choice for oatmeal and 2 more meals
- Veggies for pizza
- Chicken breast

Breakfast: Gingerbread Oatmeal
The ginger, nutmeg, and oats are all pack an anti-inflammatory punch to start your day. Adjust the spices/sweetness to your taste. Raw honey is a substitute for molasses.

- Nutmeg- .25 t
- Cinnamon- .5 t

* Ginger-.25 t
* Blackstrap Molasses- 1 T
* Water- 1.3 cups
* Steel cut oats- .25 cup

Directions:

* Boil water and put the oats in. Cover and cook until the oats are done (chewy/tender). Add in the spices and molasses with a stir.
* Take it up a notch by adding in some dried or fresh fruit. Berries and apples are good choices. If you want to add protein, consider whisking in an egg white!

Makes 1 serving

Lunch: Anti-inflammatory chickpea patties

* Turmeric ground- 1 t
* Cayenne pepper- ½ t – 1 t (depending on your heat preference)
* Sea salt- 1 t
* Potato starch- 2T
* Chickpeas- 1.5 C (usually about 1- 15 oz. can). Drain and rinse with water.
* Fresh parsley- .25 C cut roughly
* Fresh garlic- 2 cloves finely dices
* Onion, red- 1 small, diced
* Chickpea flour- appx 2 T
* Olive, grapeseed, or other cooking oil

Directions:

* Sautee the onion and garlic in a skillet with a small amount of cooking oil. Cook thoroughly on medium temperature. In the food processor, grind the chickpeas and potato starch until they reach a paste consistency. They should still have texture and not be made smooth. With short bursts, use the food processor to mix the cooked garlic and onion and the salt and pepper. Put the mixture in a bowl and incorporate the parsley.

* Spread a thin coat of chickpea flour on a flat surface. Scoop out about a ping-pong ball size ball and roll in your hand to shape into

a flattened patty. Turn the patty in the chickpea flour to coat evenly with a very light coat of flour. Repeat until all the mixture is used up.

- Heat a teaspoon of oil in the skillet on the stove over medium-high heat. Cook the patties on each side until they are browned and heated through.

- Serve on a bed of leafy green salad with a creamy avocado dressing (see day 3). Add in a wedge of melon to round out the meal.

Makes 4 servings

Dinner: Pesto Chicken Pizza

Anti-inflammatory doesn't mean you have to go without your favorites! Enjoy this pizza without damaging your body!

- Pesto:
- Pine nuts, almonds, or another roasted nut- .3 C
- Fresh Garlic- 2-3 Cloves, peeled and cut into chunks
- Basil- 2 C tightly packed (experiment with different varieties!)
- Olive Oil- .5 C
- Sea Salt- .5 t
- Lemon Juice- 1 t
- Parmesan cheese- .25 C (optional- depends on how strict you are with dairy. The recipe is fine without it!)

Directions:

Over low to medium heat and stirring constantly, toast the nuts slightly in a warm pan until hot. Place them, the garlic, basil, and cheese (optional) into a food processor. Set to a low blend and slowly drizzle in the olive oil, salt, and lemon juice. Only add enough oil to achieve a smooth consistency. You don't want soup! Store refrigerated and covered with a thin layer of olive oil over the top or freeze!

Crust/Pizza:

- Almond flour- 2 C
- Coconut oil- 2 T

- Egg (pasture raised) - 2
- Sea salt- .5 t
- Organic, pasture-raised, COOKED chicken breast- .5 lbs.
- Vegetables for toppings

Directions:

- Place the flour and salt in the bowl of a food processor and set to a low blend.

- Drizzle in the oil and then each egg until a dough forms. If still too sticky, keep adding a bit of flour a small spoonful each time.

- Form the dough into a ball (you might need to coat your fingers with flour or cooking spray to keep from sticking) and place the ball between 2 sheets of wax paper.

- Roll out until very thin- about .25 inch.

- Take off the top sheet and leave the bottom. Put on a cookie sheet. Use a fork to put a few holes throughout.

- Bake crust for 7 minutes at 350 degrees.

- Remove from oven and top with pesto, cooked chicken, bell pepper, mushroom, or whatever other pizza toppings you like!

- Return to oven and cook for another 10 – 12 minutes until the crust is fully cooked.

Serve with a side of vegetables and mixed berries for dessert!

Serves 4

Day 2
Daily Shopping List:

- Coconut water
- Pineapple
- Leafy greens
- Vegetable broth

- Parsnip
- Carrot
- Lemons/lemon juice
- Fresh Mint
- Fresh Basil
- Smoked salmon
- Asparagus
- Cabbage- red
- Rice papers
- Orange juice

Breakfast: Smoothie- Lean, green anti-inflammatory machine

- Ginger root- 1 inch
- Turmeric- .5 t ground
- Cinnamon- .5 t
- Coconut water- 1.5 c
- Pineapple chunks- 1 C frozen or fresh
- Leafy greens (your choice: kale, spinach, arugula, chard) - 2 good handfuls
- Ice if you want it thicker

Directions:

- Add everything to a blender and combine until smooth.

- Bump up the protein by adding a couple of scoops of protein powder.   Add extra some Omega-3 and other inflammation-fighting nutrients with a scoop of chia or flaxseeds.

- Makes 1 smoothie

Lunch: Carrot soup with Anti-Inflammatory Spices

- Vegetable broth- 3 C – warm
- Fresh Garlic- 4 cloves- peeled and mashed
- Onion- 1 large- cut roughly
- Parsnip- 1- peeled and cut into chunks
- Carrots- 4- peeled and cut into chunks
- Turmeric- 1t

- Fresh Ginger- 1 inch grated
- Coconut oil- .5 T
- Juice of a lemon- 3t
- Pepper and salt to your preference

Directions:

- Place freshly chopped vegetables in one layer on a baking sheet with a nonstick lining or paper.

- Sprinkle the oil over the vegetables and then sprinkle with the pepper, salt, and turmeric.

- Mix everything up a bit to make sure the oil and spices are coating all the vegetables.

- Cook 15 minutes in a 350-degree oven.
- Take them out and combine them with the warm broth, grated ginger, and lemon juice.

- Make sure you get the lid on tight! Puree on high until you have a silky, smooth consistency. Serve warm.

- To add a bit of extra flavor- add some parsley, coconut flakes or a pinch of cayenne pepper. To thin the soup or add a bit of 'cream'- consider some coconut milk.

- Serve with some whole grain crackers or toast or with a side salad of leafy greens.

Makes 4 servings

**Dinner: Salmon Asparagus Wraps
Wraps**

- Fresh Mint- .25 C chopped
- Fresh Basil- .25 C chopped
- Red cabbage- .5 C chopped or shredded
- Carrot- .5 C shredded
- Rice-paper wrappers- 6 individual 8-inch wraps

- Smoked, precooked Wild Salmon- 4 oz.
- Asparagus- .75 lbs. (about 12 average size asparagus)

Sauce

- Crushed red pepper- a pinch-1/4 t (depending on the level of heat you like!)
- Mirin (Japanese cooking wine) - 1 T (no mirin? No worries: use 1 T of rice wine vinegar and ¼ t of honey instead!)
- Juice of a lemon- 3t
- Juice of an orange- 3t
- Soy sauce- ¼ C

Directions:
Wrap:

- Bring a pan with about an inch of water to boil on the stove.

- While it is warming up- cut the bottom inch or two off the asparagus.

- Put the asparagus in the boiling water for 3 minutes or until tender.

- Remove the asparagus to ice water bath for a minute or two. Once they are cool enough to handle- remove and pat dry.

- If your asparaguses are thick, cut them lengthwise in half.

- Cut the salmon into 6 strips that will fit into the rice wrappers.

- Soak 1 wrapper at a time in hot water until it is soft (about 30 seconds). Pat it dry and place on a plate or chopping board.

- Build each wrap by putting a strip of salmon towards the bottom.

- Add a couple of asparagus spears; a little carrot, mint, cabbage, and basil. Maintain about an inch border all around the outside of the wrap.

- Start rolling at the bottom to make a tight roll and fold the sides in as you go. Cut in half to serve.

Sauce:
Combine all ingredients and mix well. Serve in a small side dish.

Serves 6

Day 3:
Shopping list:

* Almond milk
* Scallions
* Cabbage
* Cauliflower
* Bean sprouts
* Zucchini
* Avocado
* Whole grain pasta
* Lemon/lemon juice

Breakfast: Quinoa Breakfast Bowl

Harness the anti-inflammatory properties of your favorite berries and quinoa in this filling breakfast that will keep you going all day!

* Berries of choice- .5 cups
* Raw honey- 1 T
* Quinoa- .5 C cooked per package directions
* Almond milk- .5 C
* Almonds- chopped or slivers- 1 T
* Cinnamon- .25 t
* Chia Seeds- .5 t
* Zest of lemon

Directions

Combine cooked quinoa and almond milk. Stir in berries, honey, and lemon zest. Sprinkle with almonds, cinnamon, and chia seeds. Best served warm.

Serves 1

Lunch: Pad Thai in the Raw

* Bean or radish sprouts- .5 c
* Cauliflower- .5 cu
* Cabbage- purple or green- .5 c chopped
* Scallions- 2
* Carrot- 1
* Zucchini- 1

Sauce:
* Ginger Root- .5 t
* Garlic-.5 t
* Raw Honey- 1 T
* Juice of lemon- 3t
* Tahini- 2 tablespoons
* Almond (or any nut) butter- 2 T
* Soy Sauce- 3t

Directions:

* Use a spiralizer or vegetable peeler to make 'noodles' from the carrot and zucchini.

* Mix your noodles and the rest of the vegetables in a big bowl. In a small, separate dish, use a fork to mix together all of the sauce ingredients.

* Pour the sauce over the vegetables and stir, making sure everything gets an even coat.

* Let sit for at least 30 minutes but a day in the fridge does wonders for the flavours!

Makes 4 servings

Dinner: Whole Grain Pasta with Avocado Sauce

This versatile sauce is packed with vitamins and minerals that put the brakes on inflammation!   This sauce can also be used as a salad dressing or dipping sauce!

- Garlic- 2 finely diced cloves
- Green onions- 1 bunch diced
- Lemon juice- 1 lemon
- Olive oil- .25 C
- Pepper of choice and salt as you prefer
- Avocado- 2 large ripe, pitted and roughly chopped
- Whole grain pasta of your choice- about 8 oz.

Directions:

- Following the instructions on the pasta box, cook the pasta. In the food processor or blender, mix up all ingredients except the pasta.

- Using quick pulses, blend.   Once the pasta is cooked, drain- reserving .5 C of the water.

- Add the pasta water to the mixture in the food processor and blend until smooth and creamy.

- Toss with the pasta to coat and serve.   Garnish with lemon zest or a sprinkle of parsley.

Serves 4

Day 4:
Shopping list:

- Dates
- Banana
- Almond milk
- Dark Chocolate
- Tuna
- Celery
- Lime/lime juice
- Organic boneless, skinless chicken breast
- Tomato sauce

- Canned tomatoes- diced
- Canned Beans- 2 cans- black and kidney suggested
- Chili powder
- Bell pepper
- Sweet yellow onion

Breakfast: Banana Oat Muffins

Oats and ginger combine their inflammation fighting powers in this delicious muffin. With an inflammation busting kick from the dark chocolate, it is a perfect way to start the day!

- Oat Flour- 1 C *see below on how to make your own oat flour!
- Baking powder- 1 t
- Ginger- ground- .5 t
- Baking soda- .25 t
- Salt- .25 t
- Dates- .75 C pitted, chopped
- Banana- .75 C about 2 medium bananas mashed
- Almond milk- unsweetened vanilla- .5 C
- Apple cider vinegar- 1.5 t
- Vanilla extract- 1 t
- Dark chocolate- 2 T chopped into small chunks

Directions:

- Set oven to 400 degrees in temperature and spray the muffin pan with a liberal coating of cooking spray making sure you get each individual cup. In a small dish, mix the spices, baking powder and soda, and flour and place off to the side.

- Using a blender or food processor, mix dates, bananas, vanilla, almond milk, and vinegar until there are no large chunks left. Slowly add the dry ingredients to the mixture. Occasionally scrape the sides with a spatula to ensure equal mixing.

- Pour batter into a bowl, add in the dark chocolate, and stir until evenly distributed. Scoop the mixture into each muffin cup to almost full- about ¾ of the way.

- Cook muffins for about 23-26 minutes or until you can get a toothpick to come out with nothing sticky on it. Leave them to sit for about 10 minutes in the pan before you move them to a cooling rack to finish cooling off.

- Make your own oat flour: simply blitz rolled oats in a blender or food processor until they are a course flour texture.

Makes 6 muffins/servings

Lunch: Easy Tuna Salad

- Onion- 1 T finely diced
- Celery- 1 stalk finely diced
- Anti-inflammatory Mayonnaise- 1 T ** see below on how to make your own!!**
- Tuna- 1 6 oz. can water packed, drained
- Cranberries, raisins, or other dried fruit- 1-2 T
- Pepper and sea salt to taste

Directions:

- Empty the can of tuna into a bowl and add the rest of the ingredients. Stir it well and enjoy!

- For a twist- add some pickles instead of the fruit. Throw in a chopped hard-boiled egg for extra protein and other nutrients. Add in other chopped veggies like cucumber or bell pepper!

**Anti-inflammatory Mayonnaise: Combine the cream (and only the cream!) from 1 can of full fat coconut milk with lime juice (3T); olive oil (2T); Tahini or nut butter (2T); sea salt (1t) in a blender. Blend until well combined.

Makes 1 serving

Dinner: Chicken Chili (slow cooker)

- Pepper and salt as you prefer
- Cumin- 2t
- Chili Powder- 3 t

* Sweet yellow onion- 1 cut into small chunks
* Bell pepper-chopped- 1
* Fresh or canned jalapeno- 1 large fresh or 1-4 oz. can
* Fresh Garlic- 2 cloves, finely diced
* Skinless chicken breast- pasture raised- cooked and cubed- 1 lb.
* Sauce, tomato- 15 oz. can
* Tomatoes- canned, diced- 1 can with juice
* Beans- canned, black- 1 can with juice
* Beans- canned, kidney- 1 can with juice

Directions:

* Sauté onion and garlic in oil- olive or coconut- in a pan over med-high heat. Put cooked sweet yellow onion and garlic in the dish of a crockpot and put everything else in with it. Mix well. Put the crockpot on low setting for 5-6 hours (or high for 4).

* Add some garnish- try avocado slices or scallions! Serve with whole grain crackers if desired. Have an apple or some melon to round out the meal.

Serves 4-5

Day 5:
* Almond milk
* Banana
* Vegetable broth
* Lentils
* Onion
* Carrot
* Celery
* Diced tomatoes
* Baby spinach
* Avocado
* Eggs
* Fresh Basil
* Canned salmon
* Lemon juice/lemon

Breakfast: Night Before Oats

require prep on the evening before eating

- Almond milk- .75 C
- Old fashion rolled oats- .5 C
- Cinnamon- .25 t
- Chia seeds- 1.5 t
- Vanilla extract- .25 t
- Banana- 1 small, very ripe

Directions:

- Mash the banana until it is smooth and mix in the chia seeds and cinnamon.

- In a jar with tight lid, add the oats, almond milk, and vanilla. Put the banana mixture in the jar, put the lid on tightly and shake to mix all ingredients well. Leave in the refrigerator overnight and enjoy the next morning.

- Consider adding in your favorite nuts, fresh fruit, coconut flakes, a drizzle of raw honey or a few dark chocolate pieces!

Makes 1 serving.

Lunch: Tasty Lentil Soup with Spinach

Lentils are a star attraction among anti-inflammatory diet staples. These members of the legume family are high in fiber, protein, and nutrients that help prevent inflammation.

- Vegetable broth- 4 c
- Lentils- whatever color you like- 1 c rinsed and drained
- Onion- 1 large, chopped
- Carrot, peeled- 2 roughly chopped
- Celery, rinsed - 2 stalks roughly cut into small chunks
- Cloves of garlic- 2 finely diced
- Tomatoes- diced with juice- 1- 15 oz. can
- Turmeric- .5 T
- Cumin- 1.5 t
- Cinnamon- .5 t

* Cardamom-.25 t
* Bay leaf- 1 leaf
* Salt and pepper to taste
* Olive oil for sautéing- 2 t
* Baby spinach- 2 C

Directions:

* Place the cloves of garlic and pieces of onion into a big pot with a bit of cooking oil- olive or coconut preferably. Cook through and stir in carrots and celery. Cook for about 3 minutes and add turmeric, cumin, cinnamon, salt, pepper, and cardamom. Stir well and let the spices diffuse.

* Add in the tomatoes, vegetable broth, lentils, and bay leaf. Bring to a low simmer for about 18-25 minutes, or the lentils are able to be mashed with a fork. Take out bay leaf before adding the spinach and stirring it in well. Cook until it wilts.

* For a creamy soup try adding a can of coconut milk. To add brightness, try a teaspoon or two of lime juice just before serving.

Serves 4

Dinner: Salmon Patties

* Sesame oil- .5 T
* Soy Sauce- 3 t
* Raw Honey- .5 T
* Fresh Ginger- 3 t finely grated
* Lemon juice- 3 t
* Avocado- a scant .25C smashed
* Almond flour (or any nut flour) - .5 C
* Eggs- 2 (pastured raised!)
* Sea Salt- .5 T
* Salmon- 1 can 12 ounces
* Avocado Dipping sauce:
* Garlic- 1 clove peeled and chopped
* Fresh Basil- 1 handful- about .25 C chopped
* Juice of a lemon- 4 t

- Avocado- 1 large
- Olive Oil- 3 t
- Pepper and sea salt to taste

Directions:

- Combine salt, flour, salmon, and eggs in a dish and mix well using a fork. Using a separate, small dish, mix the lemon juice, honey, sesame oil, ginger, soy sauce, and avocado. Mix until smooth, add to the salmon and stir together well.

- Take about a ¼ of the mixture and form into a ball. Flatten with your hands or spatula to form a patty. Heat a heavy skillet with a teaspoon or two of cooking oil (coconut or olive oil will work). Once the oil heats, place the patties in the pan. Let them sit for a couple of minutes on each side while they turn brown and heat through.

- For the sauce: Using a blender or food processor, start with the cloves of garlic and leaves of basil until they become chopped. Put in each of the rest of the ingredients. Keep blending until there are no more chunks.

- Serve on a bed of greens and top with sauce.

Serves 4

Day 6:
Shopping list

- Carrots
- Banana
- Pineapple
- Lemon/lemon juice
- Chickpeas
- Onion
- Egg
- Wholegrain bread crumbs

* Beets
* Check for pantry ingredients

Breakfast: Anti-inflammatory Breakfast Smoothie

* Carrot juice- .5 C ** see below how to make your own**
* Almond milk- 1 C
* Banana- 1 large
* Pineapple- 1 C
* Turmeric- .25 t
* Fresh Ginger- .5 T grated
* Lemon Juice- 1 T

Directions:

* Place each ingredient in a blender and turn it on high until there are no more chunks. For a thicker smoothie- freeze pineapple and banana chunks prior to making. Add more juice for a thinner smoothie.

* ** To make your own carrot juice: place 2 carrots and 1.5 C of filtered water in a blender. Blitz on high until completely pureed. Strain through cheesecloth over a bowl. Squeeze excess juice from pulp. Store in a tightly covered jar for a few days.

Makes 1 smoothie

Lunch: Creamy Pesto Hummus

Basil is a powerhouse of anti-inflammatory properties as are chickpeas and tahini. They come together in a brilliant combination of a smooth, satisfying hummus. Look for prepared pesto that is organic and requires refrigeration to get the least processed product. Freshly made pesto is available in many delis **prepared pesto from the store will contain cheese/dairy! ** Make your own dairy-free pesto (see pesto recipe on day 1!).

* Chickpeas- 1 can
* Tahini- .25 C

* Lemon Juice- .25 C
* Olive Oil- 1 T
* Fresh Garlic- 3 cloves
* Pesto- 3 T
* Salt and pepper to taste

Directions:

* Drain the chickpeas reserving 2 Tablespoons of the juice. Combine all ingredients, including the reserved juice, in a food processor and blend until smooth. Occasionally, scrape the sides with a spatula to ensure even mixing.

* Serve with celery or whole grain crackers. Pair with a large fruit salad for a complete meal.

Makes 3 servings

Dinner:
Anti-inflammatory Beet Veggie Burger

* Onion- 1 medium, finely chopped
* Fresh Garlic- 2 cloves, finely chopped
* Egg- pasture raised- 1
* Coconut oil- .25 T in liquid form
* Whole grain breadcrumbs- 2 T
* Flaxseed- 3t
* Juice of a lemon- .5 T
* Chili Flakes- .25 teaspoon
* Sea salt- .25 teaspoon
* Beet- 2 C peeled and diced
* Olive Oil- 1 T
* Quinoa- 1 C cooked

Directions:

* Roast beets: on a cookie sheet lined with parchment paper, arrange the cubed beets tossed with olive oil in a single layer. Cook at 375 degrees for 30 minutes and set aside to cool.

* Using a food processor on pulse, puree the beets to the point that

they are mashed yet chunky.   Put the beets in a bowl.   Add in the onion, garlic, egg, breadcrumbs, flax seed, coconut oil, lemon juice, chili flakes, sea salt, and quinoa.   Mix well.   Add extra breadcrumbs if it is too moist.

* Shape mixture into 4 patties and place on a nonstick sheet for baking or use parchment paper.   Cook the burgers in the oven set to 375 degrees for a quarter of an hour.   Turn over the patties and then bake for 15 more minutes.

* Build your burger on a whole grain bun or consider the 'lettuce' bun instead.   Terrific with Avocado dipping sauce (see Salmon Patty recipe).   Pair with zucchini fries or leafy green salad for a full meal.   Try an ounce or two of dark chocolate for dessert!

Day 7:
Shopping list:

* Almond milk
* Eggs
* Avocado
* Dijon Mustard
* Mushrooms
* Frozen vegetable mix- carrots, broccoli, cauliflower (or the like) 10 oz. bag
* Onion
* Water chestnuts
* Bok choy

Breakfast: Buckwheat pancakes

* Cinnamon (optional) - 2 t
* Nondairy milk (almond works well) – 1 8oz cup
* Baking powder- 3t
* Eggs-pasture raised- 3
* Flour, buckwheat- 1.5 C
* Sea salt- .5 t
* Vanilla extract-. 5 t
* Coconut oil for cooking

Directions:

* Mix salt, baking powder, cinnamon, and flour in a dish. In a different, mix vanilla, milk, and eggs with a fork. Add into the other dish. Incorporate ingredients completely but do not over mix. The batter will be thick and lumpy.

* Heat the griddle or pan and melt the coconut oil. Spoon the batter onto the griddle and spread out if necessary. Let cook until bubbles form in the center, and the edges hold together and are dry. Use a spatula to flip to cook the other side. You will want to keep a moderate temperature in your pan as these cakes are dense and take time to cook all the way through!

* Top with fresh fruit, blackstrap molasses, raw honey, or coconut flakes.

Makes 10-12 4-inch pancakes

Lunch: Egg Salad with Avocado

Avocados are anti-inflammatory superstars! They replace the typical mayonnaise found in a traditional egg salad and add a wonderful, creamy texture. A splash of apple cider vinegar adds tang and is a trusted digestion aid.

* Pepper and salt to taste (remember- easy does it on the salt!)
* Apple cider vinegar- a splash (about .5t)
* Mustard- Dijon, coarse, or regular: .5 T
* Eggs- 3 boiled and chopped
* Avocado- .5 chopped

Smash the avocado in a bowl and add the rest of the ingredients. Stir together and enjoy!

Makes 2 servings

For a twist- add fresh or dried dill or chopped dill pickles. Serve with whole grain toast or crackers and pair with a melon salad for a satisfying meal.

Dinner: Stir Fry Asian Mushrooms

All mushrooms have anti-inflammatory properties. Asian mushrooms are particularly flavorful and go great in stir-fry. Check out your local grocery store and see what is available. Suggestions include shitake, maitake, oyster, crimini, or plain-Jane white button mushrooms.

* Mushrooms- 1.5 lbs. halved or sliced
* Frozen vegetable mix- carrots, broccoli, cauliflower (or the like) 10 oz. bag
* Coconut oil- 2-3 T for cooking
* Fresh chopped ginger- 3 t
* Fresh garlic- 2 finely diced cloves
* Onion- 1 medium chopped
* Water chestnuts (optional) - 5 oz. can drained and rinsed
* Bok choy- 1 head cut into strips
* Soy or oyster sauce- 2 T
* Egg- 1
* Quinoa- 1.5 C cooked

Directions:

* Using the directions on the box, make the quinoa and put it to the side.

* Heat the coconut oil in a skillet over medium to high heat. Once the oil is hot, start with the ginger and garlic. Cook them, stirring well, for a couple of minutes and then add in the onion. Keep stirring until the onion is translucent.

* Mix in the mushrooms until they are just beginning to brown. Stir in frozen vegetables and cook until tender. Add the water chestnuts and bok choy stirring until just heated through.

* Take the vegetable mix out of the pan and keep warm to the side. Add a small amount of oil to the pan if it is dry and then put in the quinoa and the egg. Stir the mixture until the egg is evenly mixed throughout.

- Add the vegetables back in and stir everything together. Sprinkle with soy or oyster sauce and add salt or pepper to taste.

Serves 4
CHAPTER 2: FIVE FANTASTIC BONUS RECIPES

- Add pepper and salt and the baby spinach. Stir to incorporate and serve!

- Consider adding some roughly chopped basil or parsley on top!

- For added protein, substitute chicken or fish for the chickpeas. Experiment with different vegetables and squash/pumpkins.

Makes 4 servings

Inflammation-Fighting Frittata

- Broccoli- cooked florets - 2 C chopped
- Mushrooms- 1 C sliced (any variety)
- Sweet potato- cooked- 2 C roughly cubed
- Onion- 1 medium- roughly chopped
- Fresh Garlic- 1 clove finely diced
- Eggs (pasture raised) - 6-8
- Fresh Rosemary- 1 T roughly chopped
- Fresh basil- 3 T roughly chopped
- Pepper and salt to taste

Directions:

- Steam or roast the sweet potato and broccoli and set aside.

- Cook the onion, garlic, and mushrooms in a large ovenproof skillet (season cast iron works great!) with a splash of coconut or olive oil until they are heated through, and the onions are clear.

- In a different dish, vigorously mix eggs using a whisk to the point where they are fluffy and stir rosemary, pepper, and salt.

- Put the potatoes and broccoli in the skillet and spread everything out evenly in the pan. Pour in the egg mixture and tilt the pan around to make sure the eggs are well distributed.

- Put into a preheated 400-degree oven over 8-12 minutes. Make sure the centre cooks through.
-
- Set the frittata aside for about 5 minutes before cutting to serve. Sprinkle chopped basil on top before serving.

Makes 4-5 servings.

Fish Tacos with Slaw
Anti-inflammatory Veggie Turmeric Curry

- Chickpeas- 1 can drained
- Coconut milk (full fat) - 1 can
- Baby Spinach- 2 C
- Green Peas- frozen- .5 C
- Mushroom (your choice of variety) - 1 C sliced
- Jap/Kent Pumpkin- .25 of the squash roughly chunked
- Onion- medium- 1 chopped
- Fresh Garlic- 2 cloves, peeled and finely diced
- Fresh Ginger- 1 T grated
- Coconut sugar (or raw honey) - 1 t
- Turmeric, ground- 2 T
- Coconut oil- 2T
- Pepper and salt to taste

Directions:

- Steam or roast the pumpkin until cooked and set aside.

- In a large skillet, cook oil, onion, garlic, ginger, and turmeric until the onion turns clear.

- Put the cooked pumpkin, chickpeas, mushrooms, green peas, and sugar in to cook for with the onion mixture for about 3-4 minutes.

- Add the coconut milk and stir well. Bring it to a simmer for about 15 minutes.

Slaw:
- Cabbage, red- .5 C grated
- Bell pepper, any color- .5 c sliced into very thin strips
- Onion-.25 C diced finely
- Olive, avocado, or coconut oil- .5 T
- Lime juice- 1 T (or .5 fresh lime)
- Cilantro- .25 C roughly chopped

Fish:
- Firm white fish (tilapia, cod, mahi-mahi, snapper) - 1 lb.
- Cumin- .25 t
- Cayenne pepper - .25 t (optional)
- Garlic- 1 clove finely diced
- Lime juice- 2 T (1 whole lime)
- Sea salt- .5 t

Extras: Avocado, guacamole, tomatoes or salsa

Directions:

- Combine all of the vegetables and cilantro. Sprinkle the lime juice and oil over them and toss to coat. Set aside.

- Cut the fish into bite-sized chunks. Sprinkle with spices and lime juice. Allow to sit for 15 minutes. In a nonstick/well-seasoned skillet, add about .5 T of oil and allow it to get hot on a mid-high temperature. Put the marinated fish in the skillet and move it around occasionally until it is completely cooked.

- Assemble your tacos: put 3 or 4 chunks of fish on either a whole grain tortilla or on a lettuce wrap like a large romaine or buttercrunch leaf. Top with slaw and additional garnish as desired.

Makes 4 servings.

Stuffed Portabellas with an anti-inflammatory kick

- Quinoa- 1.5 C cooked per package directions
- Organic, lean, pasture raised ground chicken or turkey- 1 lb.
- Organic salsa or diced tomatoes- .5 C
- Fresh garlic- 1 clove finely diced
- Cumin- 1 t
- Turmeric- 1 t
- Portabello caps- 4 large wiped clean and stems taken out
- Cilantro- 1 small handful roughly chopped
- Sea salt- .5 t or to taste
- Cayenne pepper- .25 t (optional)
- Olive, avocado, or coconut oil- .5 T

Directions:

- Put the cooking oil in a shallow pan and heat it over medium heat. Add in ground meat and brown. Stir in diced garlic, quinoa, and salsa. Mix thoroughly and then sprinkle with the cumin, turmeric, salt, and pepper. Stir well.

- Scoop the mixture into the mushroom caps (the stem side). Place on the selected cooking dish. Allow to cook 10 minutes at 375 degrees.

- Sprinkle cilantro on top after removing from oven. Serve with a leafy green salad with avocado dressing.

Makes 4 servings.

Anti-inflammatory balsamic grilled chicken
best if it marinates overnight!

- Basic Marinade:
- Olive Oil- .5 C
- Balsamic Vinegar- .25 C
- Dijon Mustard- 1.25 T
- Fresh Rosemary- 1 T roughly chopped
- Fresh Garlic- 2 cloves finely diced
- Turmeric, ground- 1 t
- Pepper and sea salt- .5 t each
- Organic, lean, pastured raised skinless chicken breasts- 4 breasts or about 1 lb.

Directions:

- Mix the vinegar, mustard, and herbs/spices together. Whisk in the olive oil.

- In a sealable bag, place the chicken breasts and pour in the marinade. Seal the bag and move the chicken around to make sure that they are all coated with the marinade. Refrigerate overnight.

- To cook- take the chicken out of the bag and throw it and any remaining marinade away. Put the chicken on a heated well-oiled grilling surface set to mid-range temperature. Cook about 8 minutes per side until done, and internal temperature has reached at least 165 degrees.

- Serve with wild or brown rice, quinoa, or other whole grain options and leafy green salad or roasted veggies for a healthy, filling meal full of inflammation-fighting nutrients!

CONCLUSION

Thank for making it through to the end of Anti-Inflammatory Diet - Your Guide to Eating to Minimize Inflammation and Maximize Health. Let's hope it was informative and provided you with all of the tools you need to achieve your goals, no matter what they may be.

The next step is to decide which of the tasty treats will be served first. All of them are easy to prepare with the simple guidelines provided. Why not start right now, and compile the list of everything you want to make in the first few days. You are sure to have the attention of your family when these yummy meals and snacks hit the kitchen and dining table.

With all of these new recipes, invite some friends over, and have a party. You are sure to be the hit of the neighborhood whether you choose breakfast, lunch or dinner for your menu planning. You could always have a few snacks to see if you have everyone's attention before you surprise them!

**** Remember to use your link to claim your 3 FREE Cookbooks on Health, Fitness & Dieting Instantly**

https://bit.ly/2NMfuF5

Index for Recipes

Chapter 1: 7-Day Meal Plan

Day 1:

- Breakfast: Gingerbread Oatmeal

- Lunch: Anti-inflammatory chickpea patties

- Dinner: Pesto Chicken Pizza

Day 2:

- Breakfast: Smoothie- Lean, green anti-inflammatory machine

- Lunch: Carrot soup with Anti-Inflammatory Spices

- Dinner: Salmon Asparagus Wraps

Day 3:

- Breakfast: Quinoa Breakfast Bowl

- Lunch: Pad Thai in the Raw

- Dinner: Whole Grain Pasta with Avocado Sauce

Day 4:

- Breakfast: Banana Oat Muffins

- Lunch: Easy Tuna Salad

- Dinner: Chicken Chili (slow cooker)

Day 5:

- Breakfast: Night Before Oats

- Lunch: Tasty Lentil Soup with Spinach

- Dinner: Salmon Patties

Day 6:

- Breakfast: Anti-inflammatory Breakfast Smoothie

- Lunch: Creamy Pesto Hummus

- Dinner: Anti-inflammatory Beet Veggie Burger

Day 7:

- Breakfast: Buckwheat pancakes

- Lunch: Egg Salad with Avocado

- Dinner: Stir Fry Asian Mushrooms

Chapter 2: Five Fantastic BONUS Recipes

- Inflammation-Fighting Frittata

- Fish Tacos with Slaw Anti-inflammatory Veggie Turmeric Curry

- Stuffed Portabellas with an anti-inflammatory kick

- Anti-inflammatory balsamic grilled chicken

- Basic Marinade: